THE GLUCOSE SCHOOL:

HOW TO BALANCE YOUR BLOOD SUGAR

By

GALE WATSON

Introduction

Your body uses blood sugar, commonly referred to as blood glucose, as its primary energy source. All of the cells in your body receive glucose through your bloodstream, enabling proper operation. Your body is built to maintain a steady blood glucose level. Every few seconds, the pancreas' beta cells check the level of your blood sugar. The beta cells release insulin into the bloodstream when blood glucose levels rise after eating to control the level of glucose in the blood. By acting as a key, insulin allows glucose to enter the liver, muscle, and fat cells. When your blood sugar is under control, it often goes unnoticed. However, when they fall too low or rise too high, they can interfere with your body's normal functioning.

This book is entirely devoted to glucose and how it functions within the human body. But most people aren't aware of its significance or how to manage it properly. There are a few changes you can make to your daily routine that will greatly help you if you want to manage your blood sugar levels throughout the day. You need to first understand what blood sugar spikes are and the causes of them. You must also maintain a healthy weight, eat a balanced diet rich in fruits and vegetables, and exercise frequently to prevent it.

In this book, all of these topics are covered in great detail. Let me help you start your journey to glucose enlightenment. Hope to meet you at the end.

Chapter 1

Glucose: Definition and Significance

Glucose is the most common type of sugar in the blood and the primary source of energy for the body's cells. Glucose can be created by the body from other substances or taken from the foods we consume. Another name for glucose is blood sugar. It is a monosaccharide, which is the most basic type of carbohydrate and means "one sugar."

Monosaccharides, or single sugar molecules, are often referred to as "simple" sugars. As our three primary monosaccharides, we consume fructose, galactose, and glucose. Glucose is the common link between all of these. It is a component of maltose, which is composed of two linked glucose units, lactose, which is linked to galactose, and sucrose, which is related to fructose.

Glucose is required for life in addition to being required for disaccharides. Our bodies primarily use glucose for energy, and some tissues, such as the brain, require a regular supply. Because glucose is a readily available energy source in our bloodstream, it is referred to as "blood sugar." Furthermore, the body stores it as glycogen to be used as an energy source when the blood supply of glucose is insufficient. Your body requires glucose to function properly.

What is the Source of Glucose?

The most typical monosaccharide present in nature is glucose. Photosynthesis in plants produces it. Some plants store linked chains of glucose. Starch is the name given to these chains, which are found in foods such as corn, potatoes, rice, and wheat. Some foods naturally include glucose monosaccharides, although not as a starch component. The two sources of glucose monosaccharides found in the highest concentration in whole foods are honey and dried fruits such as dates, apricots, raisins, currants, cranberries, prunes, and figs.

When glucose is extracted directly from entire foods such as apricots and dates, it is considered a natural sugar. When glucose is consumed from packaged goods and beverages to which it was added during manufacture, it is regarded as added sugar. Gluconeogenesis is the process by which glucose is created from waste products of fat and protein breakdown.

How Does Glucose Degrade?

Technically, glucose does not require digestion. Instead, it enters the bloodstream via the small intestine and is absorbed instantly, where it can be turned into energy or stored as glycogen in the liver and muscle. Before we may consume starch-containing foods, our saliva must first convert starch into maltose. The individual glucose units in maltose are then broken down further, allowing them to be absorbed. Similar to how maltose is digested, glucose is absorbed after being separated from its companion monosaccharide (galactose in lactose and fructose in sucrose). Disaccharide and starch digestion takes longer than glucose absorption, resulting in a lower blood sugar increase than ingesting glucose immediately.

Can the Body Produce Glucose?

Our bodies require glucose to function since it is used throughout the day. Given that our brain consumes approximately 60% of the glucose that our bodies ingest, this organ is critical. However, glucose does not always have to be obtained immediately through food and drink. The body manufactures its own glucose to ensure that we always have more than enough. This can be performed by dissolving glycogen to liberate the glucose it contains. Glycogen is broken down between meals and during severe activity. The gluconeogenesis process, which is mostly carried out by the liver, allows the body to produce glucose from non-carbohydrate sources. Gluconeogenesis occurs when glucose synthesis is insufficient or nonexistent, and glycogen stores are exhausted, as occurs during prolonged fasting or starvation.

The Importance of Glucose

As previously established, glucose is a universal source of energy for all living things and is also required for the human body to function properly. Glucose serves as the primary energy source for cells, particularly those in the brain, muscles, and various other body organs and tissues, as it is the fundamental fuel for energy generation. Furthermore, it promotes both aerobic and anaerobic cellular respiration. Cells receive glucose from the blood and convert it into energy molecules that they can use to perform cellular operations. During a fast, some cells, particularly those in the muscles and liver, release stored glucose. I'll go over these significances in greater depth below.

- **Brain's fuel:**

Glucose is almost totally responsible for the brain's energy requirements. It is our brain's sole source of energy for performing a variety of tasks. It is essential for neurons and the neurotransmitters they release to process signals. Because of its high energy requirements and inability to retain glucose, the brain requires a continual supply of sugar. The availability of glucose is especially important for brain neurons, which have a high metabolic rate and must use glucose as fuel in the majority of situations. The body has several defenses against extreme blood sugar drops and hypoglycemia. If there is a reduction in brain function, it is possible that brain function will fail. Some of the most common brain-related hypoglycemia symptoms are headache, dizziness, disorientation, difficulty concentrating, anxiety, irritability, restlessness, delayed speech, and poor coordination. Seizures and coma are also possible side consequences of a quick blood sugar drop.

- **Muscular power:**

Skeletal muscle accounts for about 30 and 40% of total body weight in most persons, depending on gender, age, and level of fitness. In contrast to the brain, skeletal muscle stores blood sugar as glycogen, a glucose polymer that is released during fasting. During the action, glucose is rapidly created by the breakdown of glycogen. Furthermore, muscular tissue frequently absorbs a substantial amount of glucose from the bloodstream during activity. Skeletal muscle can utilize fat molecules as an energy source, however depleting glucose reserves during prolonged activity may cause unanticipated fatigue. This is commonly referred to as "hitting a brick wall."

- **Energy for various organs and tissues:**

Different fuels can be utilized by different organs and tissues in the body. In addition to the brain and skeletal muscle, some other important organs and tissues rely on glucose as their major or exclusive fuel. A few examples from the eye include the cornea, lens, retina, red blood cells, and white blood cells. It's worth noting that, while the cells of the small intestine use glucose from food as fuel, they also largely use another molecule called glutamine. As a result, other tissues and organs that rely on sugar are left with additional glucose.

Glucose, the body's principal fuel source, helps with digestion and metabolism. It aids in nearly every element of cell metabolism, including the creation of hormones, enzymes, and energy. Following the breakdown of glucose, cells produce the energy-carrying molecule ATP. This energy-storing molecule powers nearly all of a cell's metabolic operations.

- **Structural function:**

In addition to its role in energy production, glucose is used by the human body, along with other chemicals, to generate other vital structural components. The glycoprotein collagen, for example, is composed of a protein skeleton and monosaccharides containing glucose.

Collagen is a structural polymer found in skin, muscle, bone, and other body tissues. Other glycoproteins have a substantial impact on the growth and maintenance of the body's nerves. Glycolipids, which are made up of fat and sugar components, are the foundational parts of the membrane encircling each cell in the body and its intracellular structure.

Chapter 2

Entrance into the Bloodstream: What Happens If We Don't Consume Glucose?

Glucose is largely obtained from the meals we consume. Food travels through the throat to the stomach as we eat. The stomach then begins to break it down into smaller bits with the help of acids and enzymes. During this process, our bodies convert food particles into glucose.

Glucose must cross many cell membranes to move from the digestive system, where it is found after a meal, to the body cells, where it is used. Because glucose is water soluble and cell membranes are formed of fatty material, glucose cannot cross cell membranes on its own. Insulin performs this function for it by acting as a key. It instructs cells to open so that glucose can enter. Glucose then exits the circulation and binds to a transporter protein on cell surfaces. Once it passes through the lipid barriers, the cells use or store it how they see fit.

When glucose enters our system, it goes throughout the body via the bloodstream. It exploits the circulatory system as a fuel pipeline as long as it stays in the blood. When our blood sugar levels rise or our cells need to replenish their fuel supply, glucose departs this pipeline. Our bodies attempt to maintain a consistent blood glucose level. The pancreas regulates blood sugar levels in the human body. Its beta cells check the glucose level in our blood every few seconds. When sugar levels rise, these cells release insulin.

☐ The Absorption Process

Glucose enters the bloodstream initially after absorption from the gut. Sodium-dependent hexose transporters are specialized cellular transporters that carry glucose across the digestive tract's cells. After passing through the intestinal lining, glucose is free to dissolve in the blood and move throughout the body. Because intestinal transporters operate swiftly, blood glucose levels rise rapidly after a carbohydrate-containing meal. The heart's pumping motion subsequently transfers blood glucose absorbed in the intestines to every area of the body.

☐ Cellular Intake

As the body's primary fuel source, glucose aids in the digestion of the foods we consume. It helps in practically every stage of cell metabolism, from energy production to the production of hormones and enzymes. Cells produce the energy-carrying molecule ATP once glucose is broken down. This molecule is an energy reservoir that powers practically every metabolic function in a cell.

While glucose in the bloodstream can reach all body cells, glucose entry into the cells is not as simple as it appears. Entering cells necessitates the crossing of a cell membrane, which glucose cannot do on its own. As a result, it enters the cells via particular transport proteins known as glucose transporters.

Glucose from the bloodstream enters cells with the help of two proteins. The first is known as a glucose transporter or GLUT protein. The second is the hormone insulin, which the pancreas secretes into the bloodstream to transport glucose from the blood to our cells.

Because cells require insulin to take up glucose from the bloodstream and cells require glucose to fulfill their energy needs, it is conceivable for cells to chemically "starve" even in the presence of lots of glucose if insulin is lacking. When the pancreas fails to produce insulin, cells are unable to access glucose in the bloodstream, resulting in a variety of symptoms including cellular damage and death.

☐ Glucose Transportation

There are two pathways for glucose transfer across cell membranes. A secondary active transport mechanism in which glucose is co-transported with sodium ions transports glucose against a concentration gradient in the colon and renal proximal tubule. In all other cells, glucose transport is mediated by one or more members of the closely related GLUT family of glucose transporters. The pattern of expression of GLUT transporters in distinct tissues is connected to the diverse roles of glucose metabolism in different tissues.

Carrier proteins typically transport a variety of chemicals depending on the type of cell involved. They have specialized receptors intended to recognize certain chemicals such as glucose. These proteins subsequently assist glucose in reaching our cells for usage or storage as energy. Most cells can express a variety of glucose transporters.

Glucose uptake inside our cells is typically mediated by two types of transport proteins:

Transporters that rely on sodium: This transporter type uses active transport to deliver sodium across the cell membrane. The sodium then diffuses down to carry a glucose molecule within the cell. This procedure, however, requires cell energy to move glucose across the plasma membrane.

Transporters that are sodium-independent: This transporter type does not rely on sodium to transport glucose into and out of cells. It permits glucose to enter a cell via a mechanism known as facilitated diffusion. During this process, particular proteins serve as a conduit for chemicals to breach the lipid barrier. This procedure requires no energy from the cell and transports glucose into it with minimal effort. It's as if no one entered or exited the cell.

In a nutshell, these transport proteins provide our cells with the fuel they require by transporting glucose. They also ensure that only the proper amounts of glucose enter the cell. Otherwise, glucose influxes would have impeded the metabolic activities in our cells. In the end, this may cause unwanted side effects such as inflammation or edema.

Simply said, transport proteins control glucose to keep our bodies stable.

What if There Was No Glucose in our Body?

Our body depends on glucose as a major source of energy to function properly. As fuel and a signaling molecule, glucose is a relatively prevalent metabolic substrate. Lack of glucose in our diet will cause several bodily systems to malfunction. This indicates that a reduction in the proper operation of the heart, brain, and digestive system may result from the absence of glucose in our daily diet.

Blood sugar levels can go up or down during the day depending on a variety of factors. This is commonplace. You probably won't be able to detect if it fluctuates within a specific range. However, if it falls below a healthy level and is left untreated, it can become hazardous.

Low blood sugar occurs when your blood sugar levels are so low that you must take measures to raise them to the desired range. An insulin reaction or an insulin shock are other names for low blood sugar.

 You can develop hypoglycemia if your blood glucose (sugar) level drops too low. This could be harmful and affect several body systems. Quick medical intervention is necessary. Your cells suffer from a lack of energy when your blood sugar levels are too low. Minor symptoms like hunger and headaches may first become apparent. You could face major risks if you don't raise your blood sugar levels in a timely manner.

Warning Signs and Symptoms of Low Blood Glucose

Low blood sugar has varied effects on different people. Learn how to recognize your personal low blood sugar signs and symptoms. Blood sugar levels drop after a few hours without food. In order to compensate for the lack of food, a healthy pancreas will release a hormone called glucagon. This hormone instructs your liver to release the glucose it has been holding in your bloodstream after processing them. If everything goes according to plan, your blood sugar levels should be steady until your next meal. However, not everyone experiences the signs of low blood sugar in the same manner.

By taking the time to record these symptoms, you may discover your individual signs of low blood sugar.

- A fast heartbeat and heart palpitations might result from low blood sugar levels. It takes place when you have low blood sugar so frequently that it alters how your body reacts to it. Stress hormones like epinephrine (adrenaline), the "fight-or-flight" hormone, are released when blood glucose levels are low. The hormone epinephrine is the culprit behind hypoglycemia's symptoms like a racing heart, sweating, tingling, and anxiety. These early warning signals, like hunger and shakiness, are also caused by it. Low blood sugar often indicates extreme hunger. Even if you are hungry, low blood sugar might occasionally make you disinterested in eating.

- Numerous issues with your central nervous system might result from low blood sugar levels. Weakness, dizziness, and lightheadedness are early signs. You can also experience other symptoms of stress, such as jitters, anxiety, and irritability. Low blood sugar can cause sluggishness, clammy skin, chills, and sweating. Other side effects include tingling or numbness in the tongue.

- The brain stops receiving enough glucose and ceases operating normally if blood sugar levels keep falling. As a result, one may experience impaired vision, difficulty focusing, difficulty thinking clearly, slurred speech, numbness, and sleepiness. Seizures, loss of consciousness, coma, and very infrequently death may result from prolonged blood glucose levels that starve the brain of glucose. Thus, a significant and untreated low blood sugar level might be quite harmful.

- Other symptoms may include acting or feeling irritable or hostile, headache, shaking or trembling, sweating, nervousness, foggy thinking, irritability or impatience, confusion, nausea, color draining from the skin (pallor), feeling sleepy, weak or lacking energy, coordination issues, clumsiness, and difficulty sleeping (nightmares or sobbing while sleeping).

You could still have too low blood sugar even if you are symptom-free (this is known as hypoglycemic unawareness). Until you pass out, have a seizure, or become unconscious, you might not even be aware that your blood sugar is low. Because it can harm the brain, extremely low blood sugar is a medical emergency. Checking your blood glucose levels, if possible, is the only sure way to determine whether you are experiencing low blood glucose.

Chapter 3

What You Need to Know About Glucose Spikes

Glucose, the main form of sugar in the blood, is essential for our survival. Because it maintains everything functioning properly, the body likes it as a source of energy. But like with anything, there can be too much of a good thing, and consuming too much glucose can be harmful, often without our knowledge. So, what exactly is a blood sugar spike? Here's everything you need to know.

Although "glucose spike" is not a term that is frequently used, the experience it describes is fairly likely. After consuming candy, cookies, or other sweet goodies, we experience a glucose spike, which is a momentary surge of energy. Children are particularly susceptible to this. It takes place when your blood sugar levels increase, which typically happens after a meal, an activity, or a stressful situation. Contrarily, a glucose spike is a momentary rise in blood sugar. An increase in blood sugar is both typical and expected. Glucose builds up in the blood and raises blood sugar levels, causing a blood sugar surge. When the simple sugar glucose builds up in the blood, blood sugar levels increase. However, if you regularly have spikes that are much higher than your target range, you run the risk of developing dangerously unstable blood glucose levels.

Your body will spend more time in a hyperglycemic state as a result of repeated and persistently elevated blood glucose levels. As a result, your body will experience more oxidative stress, inflammation, and glycation of crucial proteins and lipids.

Your body will produce more insulin in this situation, increasing the quantity of glucose that is taken up by your cells from the blood. Over time, if you take more insulin, your cells can become less responsive to it. As a result, your body will absorb blood glucose into your cells more slowly and you will react to insulin less effectively.

Your glucose levels increase as a result of a slower rate of glucose absorption. This can have a wide range of negative psychological and physical effects, and it may eventually cause major, potentially fatal health issues to manifest.

How Frequently are Spikes Supposed to Happen Daily?

If spikes are not too steep and stay within an appropriate range, they usually are not a problem. It is desirable to have fewer blood glucose spikes throughout the day rather than more, even if it can be challenging to totally avoid blood glucose from rising after eating or exercising. To keep your blood glucose spikes within the desired range, use proactive and preventative steps.

Blood sugar increases can last for a short while or several hours, depending on the person and even the meal. Depending on what you ate, blood sugar spikes might happen between one and two hours after you begin eating. If you consume any sugary snacks during the day, such as a chocolate bar or a piece of candy, your blood sugar levels will soar. Your blood glucose levels will increase if you consume alcohol, particularly if you drink sweet cocktails or beer that is high in carbohydrates. If you don't want to completely cut off alcohol, straight spirits or white wine are your best bets when lowering glucose spikes.

There is no cause for concern, although your blood glucose levels will undoubtedly increase after vigorous activity. Exercise encourages several advantageous glucose-spiking processes, including improved insulin sensitivity. Exercise induces stress in the body, but this tension is healthy stress.

However, you can get ready for this increase by planning your most demanding workouts for the morning or early afternoon. In this way, your blood glucose levels will have returned to normal by the time you go to bed, and your sleep won't be disturbed.

Indicators of a Blood Sugar Spike

You will experience more symptoms and your body is more prone to sustain damage the longer your blood sugar levels are high. Although there are some clear signs of high blood sugar, they differ from person to person. It's critical to recognize your unique high blood sugar signs early because doing so can prevent bodily harm from occurring. Early diagnosis and therapy could lessen the severity of the symptoms.

One of the most typical signs is fatigue. This isn't typically fatigue following a long day at work; rather, it's an irrational feeling of sluggishness while making every effort to lead a healthy lifestyle.

It is hypothesized that this sensation is caused by glucose surges. Frequent glucose surges physically overload our mitochondria, making it harder for them to adequately turn glucose into energy. As a result, human weariness is brought on by the cells' increased hunger.

Another early indicator of high blood sugar is having an extremely dry mouth, frequent urination, increased thirst, increased weariness, persistent hunger, blurred vision, lethargy, headaches, and tingling or numbness in your hands or feet. After eating, this can occur. Check your blood sugar if you encounter any of these symptoms. You can considerably help yourself regulate your blood sugar levels with something as easy as a tiny finger poke.

What Triggers a Glucose Spike?

Many factors can lead to a glucose spike. Most of the food you consume is converted to glucose. Because glucose is the main fuel for your muscles, organs, and brain to function normally, your body needs it. However, glucose must first enter your cells in order to be used as fuel.

Glucose may enter cells thanks to the hormone insulin, which is produced by the pancreas. Without insulin, glucose has nowhere to go but to float about in your bloodstream. Over time, it can become more and more focused. Blood glucose (blood sugar) levels rise as a result of the accumulation of glucose in the blood. Over time, this may harm blood vessels, nerves, and organs.

Missing insulin doses, being sedentary, and eating a lot of sugar are common causes. It's important to note that other foods can also raise blood sugar levels. Increases in blood sugar are frequently brought on by:

Diet: Diets high in sugar or carbs are more likely to cause blood sugar levels to rise than other diets. The "pizza effect" might occur while eating fatty foods. For instance, if you eat a slice of pizza, the carbs in the sauce and dough will rapidly raise your blood sugar levels, however, the effects of the fat and protein on your blood sugar levels won't be felt for several hours.

Alcohol: When combined with juice or soda, alcohol immediately raises blood sugar levels. Additionally, it may result in low blood sugar some hours later.

Sedentism: this can result from physical inactivity and raise blood sugar levels. On the other hand, intense exercise may result in physical stress, which might lead to blood sugar increases. Regular exercise is preferable to high-intensity exercise for those who have blood sugar rises. A daily regimen of exercise makes insulin work more efficiently.

Smoking: Regular blood sugar levels can be challenging to maintain while you smoke cigarettes. A smoker should prioritize stopping. Smokers may require greater insulin dosages to maintain blood sugar control.

Stress: When the body is under a lot of stress, substances are produced that boost glucose and reduce insulin's effectiveness. More glucose is therefore left in the bloodstream as a result. Finding a stress-reduction technique, like yoga or meditation, is essential.

Lack of sleep: Excellent sleep hygiene must be prioritized for some reasons. For people who experience blood sugar spikes, maintaining a consistent sleep schedule becomes essential for glycemic management. Blood sugar levels may rise as a result of sleep deprivation.

Side effects of medication: Blood sugar levels can increase as a result of some drugs. Examples of these include corticosteroids, diuretics, some blood pressure medications, and several antidepressants. Blood sugar levels may also rise as a result of taking the wrong dosage of insulin or skipping a dose.

Complications of a Blood Sugar Spike

Significant issues like heart disease, blindness, neuropathy, and renal failure are all made more likely by persistently high blood sugar levels. Diabetes and ketoacidosis can develop from untreated increased blood sugar levels. A diabetic coma or death could occur in this emergency condition. Your primary organs and bodily systems, as well as the circulation in your gums, could be harmed if your blood sugar levels stay high for an extended period of time. Some potential long-term negative effects are:

☐ **Kidney Illness**

A degenerative kidney condition called diabetic nephropathy causes the kidneys, which filter waste from the body, to stop working. It happens when high blood sugar levels harm the kidney's blood vessels. Although kidney illness may not initially show any symptoms, it might later cause renal failure.

☐ **Damage to the Nerve**

Untreated glucose spike has serious side effects, including diabetic neuropathy, or nerve damage. It results from persistently high blood sugar levels. Symptoms frequently start out mildly and worsen over the years.

☐ **Cardiovascular and Cascular Disease**

Over time, high blood sugar levels may damage the neurons and blood arteries in your heart. A blood sugar surge increases a person's chance of developing cardiovascular diseases such as heart attack or stroke.

Blood vessel obstruction could result from uncontrolled high blood sugar levels. Foot ulcers and infections may occur from this. In extreme cases, a toe, foot, or lower leg may need to be amputated.

☐ **Gum Disease**

Periodontal disease, often known as gum disease, can develop in people whose blood sugar levels rise. Increased mouth sugar can have an adverse effect on general oral health due to high blood sugar levels. Patients with high blood sugar levels have less saliva and a higher risk of developing plaque.

Blood sugar increases can result in a variety of problems, not just long-term ones. If blood glucose levels become unusually high, even briefly, quality of life suffers. Energy levels decline, mental performance suffers, physical and athletic prowess declines, and mood swings.

Remember that everything that rises must also come down. The abrupt drop in blood sugar that frequently accompanies a post-meal surge might cause false symptoms of hypoglycemia. This condition is known as "relative hypoglycemia." The brain may be fooled by the sudden change from a high to a normal blood glucose level, leading to sensations of low blood sugar. Each time there is a spike in blood sugar, some genes may be affected. This leads to the production of dangerous chemicals called free radicals, which cause inflammation and damage to the linings of blood vessels lasting hours or even days. Post-meal spikes are undoubtedly a problem worth taking into account.

Ways to Avoid Blood Sugar Spikes

It's natural for blood sugar to rise slightly after eating, but if you're continuously experiencing blood sugar spikes, assess what and how you're eating. You should visit your doctor if you're eating nutritious meals but your blood sugar levels are still rising frequently. However, by making small and simple alterations to our diets, we can keep our bodies healthy and our blood sugar levels constant.

1. Enjoy a hearty breakfast.

Since what you eat for breakfast may have an impact on your desires and hunger sensations throughout the day, think about swapping your bowl of cereal for a savory alternative like eggs to maintain levels. It is best to complement carbohydrates with protein, fiber, or healthy fats. This can assist to minimize the severity of blood sugar increases (and subsequent crashes) by slowing down the rate of glucose absorption.

2. Reduce your carb intake.

Carbohydrates cause a spike in blood sugar levels. When you consume carbohydrates, they are converted into glucose, also know as simple sugars. These sugars are subsequently delivered to the blood. When blood sugar levels rise, your pancreas releases the hormone insulin, which urges your cells to absorb sugar from the blood. As a result, your blood sugar levels plummet. Numerous studies suggest that a low-carb diet may help reduce blood sugar rises. A low-carb diet can help you lose weight and lower your blood sugar levels. You can lessen blood sugar rises by balancing your carbohydrate consumption with adequate amounts of fat and protein. Protein and fat obstruct the digestion of carbs, which keeps them from being taken into the bloodstream.

3. Consume fewer refined carbs.

Processed carbohydrates, often known as refined carbohydrates, include refined grains and sugars. Foods like table sugar, white rice, white bread, soda, candy, breakfast cereals, and desserts are examples of items that frequently contain refined carbs. Refined carbohydrates lack almost all fiber, vitamins, and minerals. Refined carbohydrates are regarded as having a high glycemic index because of how quickly and easily they are absorbed by the body. As a result, blood sugar level spikes. Whole grains, as opposed to processed grains, include the entire grain, including the fibrous bran layer on the outside and the nutrient-rich germ. When you choose whole grains, you get the most nutrients from your food. Fiber does not significantly raise blood sugar levels since it is not absorbed and broken down by the body like other carbs.

4. Put some vegetables first.

According to a new study, eating your meal in a specific order will lower the blood sugar increase that occurs from that meal by up to 75% even if you consume the same meals.2. If at all possible, eat your vegetables first. This could entail eating a side salad or the veggies from your roast dinner before a bowl of pasta. Vegetables should come first, then proteins and fats, then sugary foods and carbohydrates. Vegetable fiber coats the lining of the stomach, decreasing the rate and amount of glucose absorption, resulting in a steady rise in blood sugar as opposed to a surge.

5.   Limit Your Sugar Intake

The daily intake of added sugar in America is 22 teaspoons (88 grams). This equates to about 350 calories. The majority of it comes from prepared and processed foods like sweets, cookies, and beverages, however, some of it is added as table sugar. High-fructose corn syrup and sucrose are two extra sugars that are not required for your nutrition. In essence, they are just empty calories. These simple sugars are easily broken down by your body, which results in a quick rise in blood sugar. Consuming sugar has been linked in research to insulin resistance. Cells' inability to respond to the production of insulin prevents the body from effectively controlling blood sugar levels. Sugar is nothing but empty calories. When consumed in excess, it raises blood sugar quickly and is linked to insulin resistance.

6.   Consume more fiber

The fiber's plant-based components cannot be metabolized by your body. It can be divided into two primary categories: soluble fiber and insoluble fiber. Soluble fiber, for instance, can aid in preventing blood sugar increases. It breaks down in water to create a gel-like substance that aids in lowering the absorption of glucose in the intestines. This leads to a continuous increase and fall in blood sugar levels as opposed to a spike. Additionally, fiber might help you feel full, which will lessen your appetite and food intake. Soluble fiber-rich foods include oats, almonds, lentils, and a variety of fruits like apples, oranges, and blueberries.

7. Increase the amount of exercise you do.

Exercise reduces blood sugar peaks by raising your cells' sensitivity to the hormone insulin. Additionally, blood sugar levels are lowered through the absorption of blood sugar by muscle cells during physical exercise. It has been shown that both light and intense exercise can lower blood sugar increases. Exercise whether one is hungry or not may have an impact on blood sugar regulation. Increasing physical activity also aids in weight loss, which is beneficial on two fronts for minimizing blood sugar rises. In essence, exercise makes cells more sensitive to insulin and urges them to eliminate sugar from the blood.

8. Exercise after a meal

Walking after dinner, the largest meal of the day, can drastically lower blood sugar levels for up to 24 hours, according to research. It does not have to be a long walk because even 10 minutes of mild exercise can help lower blood sugar levels. After all, muscles use glucose as fuel.

9. Drink more water

Insufficient water intake may cause blood sugar levels to increase. Your body produces the hormone vasopressin when you are thirsty. As a result, the body is unable to remove additional sugar from your urine, which makes your kidneys retain fluid. The ideal amount of water to drink is a topic of significant debate. In the end, it is dependent upon the individual.

Drink anything whenever you feel thirsty, and increase your water intake in the summer or when you're out and about. Avoid consuming sugary beverages and juices since they will cause your blood sugar to rise. Stick to drinking water instead.

10. Keep an eye on your weight

It has been demonstrated that losing weight enhances blood sugar control. If you are overweight, your body has a harder time regulating blood sugar levels. Even a small weight loss can help you better control your blood sugar.

Blood sugar levels have wonderful impacts, but the most important thing to keep in mind is that by having a flatter glucose curve (fewer rapid peaks and dips), you may improve both your physical and mental health.

Managing Your Blood Sugar

Although glucose spikes are typical and necessary, it's important to take care to prevent a rise that is too prominent. It is critical to be able to recognize and manage high and low blood sugar levels. The most important thing you can do is consult with your doctor. Everyone has unique circumstances that necessitate a tailored plan. Here are some pointers to help you manage your blood levels properly.

☐ **Adequate water intake**

Even individuals ought to stay hydrated. Water is a component that makes up the majority of the human body and is crucial to numerous physiological functions. Water is necessary for numerous functions in life, such as digestion and nutrition absorption, joint lubrication, and body temperature regulation.

You can meet the majority of your daily fluid requirements by simply drinking water throughout the day. Water found in foods such as fruits and vegetables contributes to your daily water intake. Drinking water before and after starchy meals can also help. Choose water over sugary drinks such as soda, flavored coffee, juice, sports drinks, sweet tea, and others.

☐ **Meal schedule**

When it comes to blood sugar control, when you eat may be just as important as what you eat. A regular meal routine can assist to decrease blood sugar swings. Create a consistent eating schedule in which you eat the same amount of meals and snacks every day at around the same time. This may be five to six smaller meals spread out throughout the day, or it could be three traditional meals with two to three snacks in between. Choose an approach that works for you and stick with it.

☐ **Begin a diet and exercise plan if necessary.**

If you reduce weight, your body will be able to utilize insulin more effectively. Discuss your weight with your doctor and whether they believe lowering weight will help you reduce the probability of a spike.

☐ **Learn how to calculate your carbohydrate consumption.**

Counting carbohydrates allows you to keep track of how much you consume. Setting a limit for each meal helps to stabilize blood sugar. You can also seek for sugar-free recipes when planning your diet.

☐ **Be more active.**

Regular exercise and limiting your sitting time can help you manage your blood sugar levels. Try going for walks, enrolling in a fun exercise class, or incorporating movement into activities you currently do, such as lifting weights while watching TV.

☐ **Monitor your blood sugar levels.**

The first step in reducing blood sugar rises is to understand your blood sugar levels. You should check your blood sugar level regularly, especially if you use a medicine that directly affects it, such as insulin. Check your blood sugar level before eating every morning; this is known as a fasting blood sugar level.

The first step in addressing increased blood sugar levels in the morning is determining the cause. Checking your blood sugar before bed, in the middle of the night, and first thing in the morning can help you notice patterns in your blood glucose levels that lead to the morning high. Adhering to your medication schedule, eating a balanced diet, and engaging in regular exercise will help you manage blood sugar spikes and minimize your risk of complications.

Conclusion

Given the multiple benefits of blood glucose control, starting to measure and assess your after-meal management is undoubtedly worthwhile. If your blood glucose levels are higher than they should be, talk to your doctor about new or modified medical treatments. Also, examine your personal food and exercise choices. Even without a completely working pancreas, there are numerous ways to manage those high blood glucose spikes!

Chapter 4

Why Do I Crave and Consume More Glucose Than Needed?

The term "craving" refers to an intense desire for a particular food. Cravings may also be your body's way of alerting you that it isn't obtaining a necessary nutrient, such as a particular vitamin or mineral. Cravings are common and can vary in intensity and frequency depending on a number of factors. On the other side, blood glucose imbalances usually cause sugar cravings. It's possible that you need something sweet to increase your blood sugar levels.

We have a natural tendency to seek sweets, to some level. Our brains have evolved to enjoy sweet foods because glucose is a vital fuel source for our bodies. Our brains adapt to need more sugar to provide the same pleasurable experience when we regularly consume sweet meals. In other words, you become more addicted to sugar the more you consume. It has been discovered that sugar makes the brain more prone to addiction. In fact, immediately cutting it out of your diet may cause withdrawal symptoms like drowsiness, depression, headaches, and muscle aches.

Another way to look at it is to think about how your body uses sugar to raise blood sugar levels, which then causes your body to release insulin to lower the level to a safe level. When insulin lowers blood sugar levels, as it frequently does, the body looks for ways to raise them and increase energy.

You could be putting yourself at risk for a wide range of detrimental health effects if you give in to this temptation too frequently. All that extra sugar has the potential to boost caloric intake and fuel chronic inflammation. You don't have to completely deprive yourself of the foods you want, though. The idea is to figure out why you crave them and to make sure your diet is balanced and nutritious overall. Eat foods that stop too much insulin from being released, such as protein and healthy fats, and take in very little sugar to control your blood sugar levels.

Why Do We Have Sugar Cravings?

There are patterns in your eating plan that cause you to crave sugary foods. One example is poor protein intake. Because protein and fats limit the release of sugar into your bloodstream, if you don't consume enough of them, your blood sugar can increase and fall at an irregular rate. This explains why a diet strong in carbohydrates may make you crave sweets. Quickly absorbed simple carbs increase blood sugar and insulin levels by speeding up their absorption into the body. You won't feel satisfied or full with simple carbohydrates alone, and you'll start to crave more.

Surprisingly, your body desires the quick energy it is used to when you stop eating carbohydrates. The first few days of a low-carb diet are usually marked by a high-sugar craving. Once your body adjusts to functioning without carbohydrates, the hunger disappears. Increasing your protein consumption is simple with a high-quality protein powder.

- **Habitual Actions**

It turns out that long-term programming is frequently the cause of sugar cravings. To put it another way, it's a habit. A stimulus triggers a behavior, which is followed by a reward. This may sound perplexing, so allow me to clarify. The hormone that makes us feel happy after eating our favorite dessert is dopamine, whereas the hormone that controls blood sugar levels is insulin (also known as the stimulation hormone). The primitive brain regions that act as our reward pathway experience an increase in insulin levels when we consume sugar (the activity). Dopamine is released in response to this, which makes us feel good (the reward) and causes us to become accustomed to eating sugar. This causes our bodies to start associating eating sugar with happiness and the want to keep eating sugar in order to feel happy, which can culminate in a cycle of pleasure-seeking. Our upbringing may also contribute to the development of a sweet tooth. Maybe you watched your parents overindulge on Thanksgiving when you were younger, and now you do the same thing, eating pies in excess even when you are not hungry. Maybe you've spent years looking for chocolate to make you feel better or ice cream to make you feel happier. Determine what is driving your cravings, whether it be a habit, emotional eating, or true hunger, by paying attention to them.

- **Low Levels of Serotonin**

If you've ever wondered why you might feel the need to overindulge in desserts like ice cream after a trying day, your serotonin levels may play a role. When we are anxious, upset, or sad, our bodies seek serotonin because it helps to regulate mood. According to research, the onset of depression may be influenced by serotonin imbalance in the brain.

You are typically drawn to foods that promote the creation of serotonin while you are wanting carbohydrates. Sugar cravings as well as some other symptoms like mood disorders, anxiety, and sleep difficulties have all been connected to low levels of the neurotransmitter serotonin. It is commonly recognized that serotonin influences mood, general emotions of well-being, and the regulation of appetite and food intake.

In a way, we turn to sugary, carbohydrate-rich foods as a coping mechanism for depression. You may take control of your cravings rather than allowing them to rule you by being more knowledgeable about the relationship between food and emotion.

- **Stress and Insufficient Sleep**

Stress is among the most frequent causes of overindulgence in sweets. When you are under stress, your body produces a lot of the hormone cortisol, which causes your liver to release glucose, raising your blood sugar. Stress can frequently lead to an increase in both appetite and cravings, but it does so in different ways for different people. When under intense stress, cortisol levels are high, which contributes to the well-known feeling of being in overdrive. While operating at full capacity, your body will quickly exhaust its energy reserves and look for quick ways to restock them. Because we are aware that blood sugar swings can lead to cravings, being under constant stress is like asking for a spike.

Your desire for sugar may also be caused by a lack of sleep. The hormones ghrelin and leptin, which encourage and inhibit food intake, are significantly controlled by your sleep-wake cycle. Short sleep periods cause these hormones to become unbalanced, which increases appetite and decreases feelings of fullness. The cerebrum, the area of the brain responsible for making complex judgments and decisions, has been shown in studies to be negatively impacted by even one night of poor sleep. Overeating, especially the overconsumption of sugar and junk food, can also be brought on by a lack of sleep. Because of this, consistently experiencing irregular sleep patterns or sleep deprivation can have a serious negative impact on your health.

Sugar consumption is also a physiologically adaptive behavior that gives people the energy they need to stay awake. Sugar is a soluble carb, and we are hardwired to seek them when we are stressed. Sugar is also the first thing we seek when we are tired or exhausted because it is the body's primary source of energy and it is quickly digested.

- **Mineral Deficits**

According to our belief, if your body yearns for a certain flavor or food, you must be deficient in that substance. That may be true in the majority of situations, as in the case of salty foods and sodium deficiency. However, in certain instances, the hunger for sweet, sugary foods may be caused by specific mineral imbalances in the body.

You will feel exhausted and weak as a result of an iron shortage. To wake yourself up, your body will need rapid energy, which may help to explain why you have a sweet tooth. Unbalances in calcium, zinc, chromium, and magnesium can also cause sugar cravings. Together, these minerals play a vital role in hundreds of bodily functions, including the metabolism of carbohydrates and the production and management of the hormones and enzymes that influence your thoughts, feelings, and movements. You can be having unusual reactions to the thought, sight, or smell of anything sweet if you aren't getting enough of these minerals to consume, absorb, and store.

- **Your meal was not balanced.**

You overate on carbohydrates and underate on fat, protein, or both. You almost certainly set yourself up for a guaranteed gelato yearning when you consume a heavy, starchy dinner like a huge dish of spaghetti. All that pasta devoid of fiber or protein is equivalent to a large bowl of sugar, which can cause a blood sugar rise and fall and leave you craving more sugar. Because they are quickly absorbed, the calories in that bowl of spaghetti don't make you feel full or pleased.

- **Misread signals**

Our bodies occasionally interpret brain messages incorrectly. For instance, the body may start to indicate hunger when it is thirsty, and we may misinterpret this as a desire for sugar. In other situations, we could require a boost in energy, so we turn to a candy bar for a temporary solution.

- **You snacked on lots of salty foods.**

Your food contains more sodium than you probably even realize when you eat out or consume highly processed, packaged foods. In most cases, this holds even if you order grilled salmon or steamed spinach from a restaurant of your choice. The worst part is that you frequently crave sweets more when your diet is saltier.

In conclusion, even as we become older, we still tend to love sweets, though less so. Each person's level of preservation of that preference is unique and appears to be influenced by a variety of factors, including living circumstances. The dread of a spike, however, does not need you to completely eliminate sweets from your diet. Although you can still consume it in moderation, it's crucial to read labels before you purchase because hidden sugar may be present in items you wouldn't expect. The quantity of sugar you consume can significantly change by making a few healthy substitutions.

Chapter 5

Keeping Your Blood Sugar in Check

There are several ways to lessen or manage the way your body's glucose levels spike. All that is necessary is a modification in your everyday routine, and the results you get will be beneficial to your health.

1. Follow the right eating sequence.

People may feel constrained or overwhelmed by the idea of consuming only foods that balance their blood sugar. But there's more to preventing unnecessary glucose surges than just what you eat. Some of us like to keep our favorite foods for last, while others like to eat them first. Did you know, however, that merely switching the order in which we consume our meals may have an impact on our blood sugar levels? Timing your carbohydrate intake may also aid in blood sugar management and weight maintenance, both of which will support your overall health objectives. As a result, the order in which the foods on the plate are consumed has a big influence on how much glucose and insulin are produced after eating.

It's not necessary to restrict your strategic eating for blood sugar balance to the items you eat. As you can see, meal pairing is governed by several rules. On the other side, eating in order is significantly simpler. It's less about meal combos and more about eating in the right order. You can prevent a blood sugar spike by eating your meals in a specific order, and this tip works with any meal. Consuming your meals in a certain order is one method that doesn't involve limiting your food options.

The ideal order for ensuring constant blood glucose levels is vegetables first, followed by proteins and fats, and last, carbohydrates and sugars. This arrangement of foods reduces the rise in blood sugar and its associated negative consequences by up to 75%. Compared to eating the same things in the reverse order, starting a meal with vegetables and protein and ending it with carbohydrates will keep you fuller for longer. This is because protein delays the bloodstream's absorption of sugar from carbohydrates, preventing a spike in sugar followed by a decline. Lower post-meal glucose and insulin levels are the outcomes of consuming protein and veggies before carbohydrates. The timing of carbohydrate consumption is more important than the quantity.

To be more precise, try having something substantial and savory for breakfast rather than anything sugary. For lunch and dinner, for instance, start with greens like broccoli and fats like avocado or almonds rather than adding eggs and vegetables to your meal to maximize your micronutrient intake. Dessert comes last but not least. Eat a snack of starchy carbohydrates, like a banana, along with a source of protein, fat, or fiber to control post-meal hyperglycemia. You'll be more balanced throughout the day if you have less sugar in the morning. Plan your meals in advance to prevent blood sugar drops.

Protein is rich in satiety and keeps you full for a long period, whereas salads and vegetables are high in fiber and minerals and can quickly fill you up. We frequently consume carbohydrates first since they are the most delectable macronutrient. While carbohydrates are generally not bad for you, every meal needs to have enough protein and fat. Blood sugar levels can be affected by sugary beverages like sweetened tea. Make a sweet beverage a reward after your meal rather than drinking it sooner if you wish to include it.

2. Avoid an Early-Morning Spike

The notion that eating something sweet for breakfast is healthy because it gives us energy is a common fallacy. Though eating something sweet makes us happy, it's not the best approach to get energy, so this statement is untrue. A standard bowl of cereal may cause blood sugar levels to rise. Corn or wheat kernels that have been processed are used to make cereal. Nothing but starch; there is no fiber. Table sugar is added to the mixture because starch isn't the most enticing ingredient by itself. Minerals and vitamins are added to the mixture, but their benefits do not outweigh the negative effects of the other ingredients.

Additionally, our bodies are most vulnerable to glucose when we first wake up and are empty-handed. Since our stomachs are empty, anything that enters them is processed very rapidly. As a result, eating sugars and carbohydrates for breakfast frequently causes the day's biggest gain. Even though breakfast is the worst meal of the day to consume primarily sugar and carbohydrates, most people nevertheless do it. Training oneself to eat savory breakfasts rather than sweet ones are preferred.

The good news is that some foods, especially at the start of the day, can help regulate blood sugar levels. Here are some of the best breakfast foods for controlling or even lowering blood sugar.

Proteins and fats: You may have heard that increasing the amount of protein and fat in your diet will aid with blood glucose regulation. Additionally, protein and fat restrict the movement of food through the digestive system, which lowers the quantity of glucose released into the circulation when carbohydrates enter the body. Protein and fat can be found in chicken, fish, pig, eggs, beans and peas, butter, oils, avocado, Greek yogurt, tofu, cheese, cream cheese, and other dairy products. In addition to being a great source of protein, nuts and seeds are frequently seen in a balanced meal. Chemicals found in nuts help keep insulin and glucagon, two hormones important for controlling blood sugar, in balance. So it's a great idea to include a variety of healthful nuts and seeds in your diet. For stabilizing blood sugar levels, try almonds, cashew nuts, pistachios, peanuts, walnuts, flaxseeds, and pumpkin seeds.

Fiber: Getting enough fiber in the morning might be difficult because it necessitates eating salad and vegetables for breakfast. Fiber forms a net in the upper intestines, keeping the body from absorbing too much glucose from the meal's remaining components. Chia seeds are an excellent example of a high-fiber diet that can help to mitigate the consequences of glycemic responses. They contain a lot of protein, antioxidants, healthy fats, and fatty acids like omega-3s, all of which have been linked to better blood glucose management in some way.

Monitoring and tracking your blood glucose levels may appear tough, but it does not have to be. Making dietary and lifestyle adjustments is one of the most effective ways to reduce blood sugar spikes. If you guarantee that your blood sugar levels are healthy when you get up, you can easily advance and reach your health goals throughout the day. A nutritious breakfast is also a great way to start the day.

3. Instead of a snack, opt for a dessert.

People may find it difficult to distinguish between a dessert and a snack. Dessert is the concluding course of a meal. It comprises foods such as desserts and fruits, as well as beverages such as wine or liqueur. It could include coffee, nuts, pudding, ice cream, and other delectable savory goodies. A snack is something you eat in between meals or for a few hours after dinner. Fruit, yogurt, cookies and milk, or cheese and crackers could be served as a snack. A slice of cake or pie is another choice.

The fundamental contrast between desserts and sweets is how they are presented or consumed. Candy can be had at any time, however, sweets such as cakes, pastries, and ice cream should be savored and devoured after a meal. When you eat something, rather than what it is, defines whether it is a dessert or a snack.

Remember to eat your meals properly and save the sweet treat for dessert at the end of the meal if you find yourself needing something sweet during the day. If you must snack, go for something savory. Some ideas include a hard-boiled egg, veggies, crackers and cheese, dark chocolate, and yogurt topped with chopped almonds.

4. Watch Out for Unexpected Sugar Sources

You're probably aware that sugary foods, baked goods, and drinks can all elevate blood sugar levels. However, even if it does not taste sweet or include additional sugar, anything heavy in carbs has the potential to have a comparable effect. Avoid eating too much refined bread and cereals that have been heavily processed.

Along with many plant-based milk alternatives, bottled salad dressings and condiments such as ketchup and barbecue sauce typically contain an unexpectedly high sugar content. Always read labels before buying any product. Fruit is another example, especially if you choose dry fruit or offer large servings. Although whole fruit is normally preferred, high-sugar fruits such as grapes, bananas, melons, and mango should be avoided in excess.

5. After your meal go for some exercise.

It is normal for your blood sugar levels to momentarily rise after eating a meal, particularly one high in carbohydrates. Glucose from the intestine enters the bloodstream after a meal, raising blood sugar levels.

Moving shortly after eating, such as taking a stroll, causes your heart rate to slightly increase and you breathe harder. Muscle tissue quickly absorbs the glucose in our blood, lowering blood sugar levels.

Simply put, when you exercise, your heart pumps more glucose-containing blood to your muscles, your muscle membranes become more effective at absorbing glucose, and changes in chemical enzymes promote even greater glucose transfer. As a result of all of these mechanisms working together to provide our muscles with the glucose they need to accomplish a workout, our blood glucose levels fall.

More importantly, exercise allows muscle tissue to absorb glucose without the need for insulin, whereas the body ordinarily releases insulin to transport glucose into cells. Because we aim to keep insulin levels as stable as possible, lowering the quantity of insulin produced in response to glucose increases after meals is beneficial. Insulin resistance can develop as a result of elevated insulin levels over time.

Blood sugar levels can be controlled by avoiding long periods of sitting during the day, consuming nutritious foods, and maintaining a healthy weight. Even if it's only for a few minutes, going for a short walk after eating can help drop blood sugar levels. The duration of your exercise, among other factors, will impact how your physical activity affects your blood sugar levels. It's crucial to note that exercise might cause a reduction in blood sugar for up to 24 hours or more thereafter. Remember that you don't have to go overboard. Blood sugar levels may temporarily rise after indulging in vigorous activity. Excessive exercise can elevate stress hormone levels, which can raise blood sugar levels.